VANESSA ROSE

The Diabetic Diaries

A Young Adult's Guide To Navigating Type 1 Diabetes

Contents

1 Owning Your Diabetes Journey   1

2 What is Type 1 Diabetes   2

3 The Highs and Lows   5

4 Building Your Diabetes Team   9

5 Navigating Everyday Life   12

6 The College Years: Managing Diabetes Independently   16

7 Relationships, Dating, and Type 1 Diabetes   21

8 What Happens When Things Go Wrong   24

9 Celebrating Success and Living Your Best Life
With Type 1   27

10 Conclusion: You've Got This!   31

11 Resources   33

Epilogue   35

1

Owning Your Diabetes Journey

Dear Diary: DIABETES? Really?!

"Owning your diabetes means taking control—not just of your blood sugar levels, but of your story."

When you first get diagnosed with Type 1 Diabetes (T1D), it can feel like the world has flipped upside down. Suddenly, your body isn't quite the same, and every day involves making choices—about food, exercise, insulin, and more—that affect your health. In many ways, it can feel like diabetes is something that's happening *to* you rather than something you have any control over. It can feel like you're simply responding to the disease, playing catch-up with your body's needs.

But what if I told you that owning your diabetes journey means transforming that narrative? Instead of just reacting, you can begin to *drive* the story of your life with diabetes. While the disease itself will always be a part of you, how you live with it—and how you shape your response to it—is entirely in your hands.

2

2

What is Type 1 Diabetes

Dear Diary: So apparently I have Type 1 Diabetes now. I thought only old people had diabetes.. I guess it's time to Google my new best friend. Great.

Type 1 Diabetes (T1D) is a chronic autoimmune condition in which the body's immune system mistakenly attacks and destroys the insulin-producing cells in the pancreas called beta cells. Insulin is a hormone that helps regulate blood sugar (glucose) levels, allowing the body to use glucose for energy. Without sufficient insulin, glucose builds up in the bloodstream, leading to high blood sugar (hyperglycemia), while the body's cells are starved for energy.

Unlike Type 2 Diabetes, which is often linked to lifestyle factors and insulin resistance, Type 1 Diabetes is not preventable and typically develops in childhood or adolescence, although it can be diagnosed at any age. It is often referred to as an autoimmune disease because the body's immune system mistakenly attacks the pancreas cells responsible for producing insulin (Atkinson et al., 2014). This autoimmune response is still not fully understood, but researchers believe that genetic and environmental factors, such as viral infections, may trigger the onset of T1D in genetically predisposed individuals.

The symptoms of T1D can develop quickly and include excessive thirst, frequent urination, fatigue, blurred vision, and unexplained weight loss. If left untreated, high blood sugar can lead to dangerous complications, such as diabetic ketoacidosis (DKA), a potentially life-threatening condition that occurs when the body starts breaking down fat for energy due to the lack of insulin, producing acidic byproducts called ketones.

How Is Type 1 Diabetes Managed?

Managing T1D involves a lifelong commitment to regulating blood sugar levels through a combination of insulin therapy, diet, exercise, and regular blood sugar monitoring. Insulin is typically administered through multiple daily injections or via an insulin pump. The goal is to mimic the natural insulin release that would occur in a non-diabetic pancreas, adjusting doses based on food intake, activity levels, and blood sugar readings.

A key component of T1D management is blood glucose monitoring, which is usually done multiple times a day with a glucometer, or for some, through continuous glucose monitoring (CGM) systems that provide real-time glucose data. Managing T1D can be challenging, requiring constant attention and adjustments, but with the right tools and education, most individuals with T1D can lead healthy, active lives.

Prevalence and Impact

T1D is less common than Type 2 Diabetes but still affects millions worldwide. In the United States, about 1.6 million people are living with T1D, and more than 200,000 children and adolescents are diagnosed with the condition (Centers for Disease Control and Prevention [CDC], 2022). The impact of Type 1 diabetes extends beyond the physical, as managing a chronic condition from a young age can lead to emotional challenges like stress, anxiety, and worries about long-term health complications.

3

The Highs and Lows

Dear Diary: I swear, some days, having T1D feels like being a contestant on a game show that I wasn't told the rules on how to play.. Oh and the host is speaking Chinese. What in the world is going on?? I swear, my emotions are more unpredictable than my glucose levels.

Living with Type 1 Diabetes (T1D) is a constant balancing act—one that can affect not only the body but also the mind. Managing blood sugar levels, adjusting insulin doses, monitoring food intake, and planning exercise can create a significant emotional burden, especially for those who are newly diagnosed or navigating the complexities of T1D throughout their lives. The emotional toll of diabetes management is often underestimated, but it can have a profound impact on mental health and overall well-being.

Stress and Anxiety

One of the most common emotional challenges for people with T1D is diabetes-related stress. This stress arises from the daily demands of managing the disease, constantly checking blood glucose levels, making decisions about food, exercise, and insulin, and the fear of potential complications (e.g., hypoglycemia or diabetic ketoacidosis). The unpredictability of blood sugar fluctuations adds to this stress, as even the most carefully planned day can be disrupted by unforeseen highs or lows.

In fact, studies have shown that people with T1D experience higher levels of anxiety compared to the general population. Diabetes-related distress (a form of stress specific to living with diabetes) can contribute to feelings of helplessness and burnout, as individuals struggle to meet the constant demands of self-care (Cameron et al., 2008). For young adults, the stress of managing diabetes while balancing school, work, relationships, and social activities can be particularly overwhelming.

Depression

Living with a chronic illness like T1D also increases the risk of depression. According to research, individuals with T1D are more likely to experience symptoms of depression than the general population, and those with poorly controlled diabetes may face an even greater risk (Anderson et al., 2001). Depression can make it even more difficult to manage diabetes effectively, as feelings of fatigue, sadness, or hopelessness may reduce motivation to maintain regular blood sugar monitoring, adhere to insulin regimens, or make healthy lifestyle choices.

Diabetes Burnout

Another emotional challenge that many people with T1D experience is diabetes burnout. This term refers to the emotional exhaustion and frustration that can arise from the constant vigilance required in managing the disease. Over time, some individuals may feel overwhelmed by the relentless cycle of diabetes care, leading to neglect of their health and a sense of disengagement from their treatment plan (Pouwer et al., 2010). Burnout can manifest as feelings of frustration, resentment, or a sense of defeat, which can negatively impact both mental health and diabetes management.

Strategies for Coping

While the emotional challenges of living with T1D are real, there are strategies to help manage the emotional toll. Mental health support, such as therapy or counseling, can provide a safe space for individuals to process their feelings about living with a chronic illness. Support groups, both in-person and online, allow people with T1D to connect with others who understand their experiences. Additionally, practicing self-compassion and setting realistic expectations for diabetes management can help reduce feelings of guilt or frustration.

Ultimately, recognizing the emotional side effects of T1D and addressing them proactively is crucial for long-term mental and physical health. By acknowledging and managing these challenges, individuals with diabetes can build a more balanced and empowered approach to living with the condition.

4

Building Your Diabetes Team

Dear Diary: Apparently, managing diabetes requires a whole team. So today I started the hunt for my squad—doctor, dietitian, maybe a therapist if they can handle my 2 a.m. panics. Fingers crossed I find the Avengers of diabetes care.

Managing Type 1 Diabetes (T1D) is not a solo endeavor. One of the most important factors in achieving successful diabetes management is having a strong, supportive team of healthcare professionals, family members, and peers who work together to help you navigate the challenges of living with T1D. Building a successful diabetes team means surrounding yourself with individuals who understand your needs, provide expert guidance, and offer emotional support.

Key Members of Your Diabetes Team

1. **Endocrinologist**: As the primary healthcare provider for individuals with T1D, an endocrinologist specializes in hormone-related conditions, including diabetes. They will help you manage insulin therapy, adjust your treatment plan, and monitor your long-term health.
2. **Diabetes Educator**: A certified diabetes educator (CDE) provides education on managing blood sugar, insulin use, nutrition, and lifestyle changes. They can help you develop the skills necessary to manage your diabetes day-to-day.
3. **Dietitian**: Nutrition plays a critical role in managing diabetes. A registered dietitian can help you create a personalized meal plan that aligns with your insulin regimen and lifestyle.
4. **Mental Health Professionals**: Living with a chronic illness like T1D can be emotionally taxing. A therapist or counselor can help

you address diabetes-related stress, anxiety, or depression and develop coping strategies.

5. **Family and Support System**: Having a network of family and friends who understand your condition and offer emotional support is essential. They can encourage you to stay on track with your diabetes care and help you stay positive.

Collaborative Care

A successful diabetes team works collaboratively, with everyone on the same page. Regular communication between team members ensures that adjustments to your care plan are made when necessary, and that you are supported in all areas of your health—physical, emotional, and social.

Having a reliable, experienced team can empower you to manage your diabetes more effectively and improve your overall quality of life.

5

Navigating Everyday Life

Dear Diary: This morning, I seriously considered throwing all my diabetes management out the window and eating an entire pizza (deep dish to be exact). But then, like a responsible adult - with a smidge of self-discipline, I opted for a salad and a jog instead. I'm not saying I didn't cry a little inside, but at least I avoided a carb coma.

Living with Type 1 Diabetes (T1D) means integrating diabetes management into nearly every aspect of your daily life. It requires making constant decisions about insulin, food, exercise, and stress levels, all of which can influence blood sugar levels. While managing diabetes may feel overwhelming at times, with the right tools and knowledge, you can successfully navigate the challenges of daily life.

Managing Blood Sugar Levels

Blood sugar (glucose) management is at the core of living with T1D. Since the body no longer produces insulin, individuals with T1D must rely on insulin therapy to help regulate blood glucose levels. Blood glucose levels need to be monitored regularly, typically multiple times a day, using a glucometer or continuous glucose monitoring (CGM) system. CGMs offer real-time data, making it easier to detect trends and respond to changes in blood sugar before they become problematic.

It's essential to adjust insulin doses based on factors like carbohydrate intake, physical activity, and stress levels. For example, insulin doses may need to be increased after consuming meals rich in carbohydrates, while physical activity may lower blood glucose levels, requiring a reduction in insulin or an increase in carbohydrate intake to prevent hypoglycemia (low blood sugar).

Diet and Food Choices

What you eat plays a crucial role in blood sugar management. Unlike Type 2 Diabetes, which is often managed through lifestyle changes alone, individuals with T1D must still manage insulin doses based on the foods they eat. Understanding how different foods affect blood sugar is key to maintaining stable levels. Carbohydrate counting is an essential skill for individuals with T1D. Foods that contain carbohydrates, like bread, pasta, fruit, and sugary drinks, are broken down into glucose, which can cause blood sugar spikes. By counting carbs and adjusting insulin accordingly, you can keep your blood sugar levels within a target range (American Diabetes Association, 2023).

Choosing nutrient-dense foods that have a lower glycemic index (GI)—meaning they cause slower, more gradual increases in blood sugar—can help stabilize blood glucose levels throughout the day. Whole grains, vegetables, lean proteins, and healthy fats are good options for managing diabetes (Ludwig, 2002).

It's also important to maintain portion control, as overeating can lead to larger insulin doses, which may cause blood sugar swings. The American Diabetes Association suggests a balanced approach to meals, focusing on vegetables, lean protein sources, and high-fiber carbohydrates to avoid large fluctuations in blood glucose levels.

Exercise and Physical Activity

Exercise has a profound effect on blood sugar levels, often lowering them. Regular physical activity helps improve insulin sensitivity, allowing the body to use insulin more efficiently. However, exercise can sometimes lead to hypoglycemia, particularly if insulin doses aren't adjusted properly before or after physical activity. It's important to monitor blood sugar levels before, during, and after exercise, and carry a quick source of glucose, such as juice or glucose tablets, in case of a drop in blood sugar (American Diabetes Association, 2023).

Stress and Its Effect on Blood Sugar

Stress—whether due to work, school, relationships, or other factors—can also impact blood sugar levels. Stress hormones, such as cortisol, can increase blood sugar levels, making it more difficult to maintain stable glucose levels. Managing stress through techniques like mindfulness, yoga, or deep breathing exercises can help reduce its impact on diabetes control (Anderson et al., 2001).

Sleep and Blood Sugar

Adequate sleep is another key factor in managing diabetes. Poor sleep can lead to insulin resistance and higher blood sugar levels the following day. Establishing a consistent sleep routine and aiming for 7-9 hours of sleep per night can support better blood sugar control.

Building Healthy Habits for Long-Term Success

Living with T1D requires making decisions and adjustments every day, but with a proactive mindset and the right support, it becomes more manageable. The most successful approaches involve a combination of self-monitoring, education, and healthy lifestyle choices—all of which help you maintain control over your blood sugar and live an active, fulfilling life.

6

The College Years: Managing Diabetes Independently

Dear Diary: When I said I wanted to take shots at the bar, insulin is not exactly what I meant. Oh and some girl just mistook my insulin pen for a vape. No, I'm NOT kidding.

The transition to college is a major milestone, filled with new opportunities, challenges, and independence. For young adults with Type 1 Diabetes (T1D), this period presents unique hurdles that require a delicate balance of self-management, personal responsibility, and social interactions. Navigating the complexities of managing diabetes while adjusting to college life can be overwhelming, but with the right strategies and support, students with T1D can thrive both academically and socially.

Navigating Independence

One of the most significant changes when moving to college is gaining independence. For many, this means taking full responsibility for managing their T1D, from administering insulin to monitoring blood sugar and maintaining a healthy diet. The freedom of managing your own schedule can be empowering, but it also requires careful planning and discipline.

Without the structure provided by parents or caregivers, it's important to develop a routine for diabetes management. This includes setting aside time for blood sugar monitoring, insulin injections or pump management, and meals. Using tools like diabetes management apps can help students track their blood sugar levels, insulin doses, and carb intake, making it easier to stay on top of their care (Diabetes Technology Society, 2020). Additionally, keeping a diabetes kit in a convenient, easily accessible place (such as a backpack) with supplies like insulin, a glucometer, extra snacks, and a glucagon kit is essential for emergencies.

Students should also consider informing their college health center about their diabetes. Many colleges have health services that can provide support in managing diabetes, including regular check-ups, assistance with prescriptions, and educational resources. Some schools may also offer accommodations, such as extended time for exams or permission to eat during class, which can help manage the day-to-day demands of diabetes care.

Dealing with Social Situations

College life brings an abundance of social opportunities, including dining with friends, attending parties, and participating in extracurricular activities. However, for students with T1D, these social situations can present challenges when it comes to managing blood sugar levels and staying on track with diabetes care.

Dining out with friends or choosing meals from a cafeteria can be tricky, especially when you have limited control over the food preparation. Carb counting and making smart food choices are essential skills for managing blood sugar levels. Communicating your dietary needs to friends or waitstaff can be helpful in avoiding high-carb or high-sugar options. Many campuses offer meal plans with healthy, diabetes-friendly options, so taking time to plan meals can make navigating these situations easier.

Social gatherings, such as parties, barbecues, or late-night events, may present more complex challenges, particularly when it comes to consuming food and alcohol. Maintaining your blood sugar within a healthy range can be difficult if your eating and activity patterns vary from your usual routine. Prioritizing balanced meals, bringing your own diabetes-friendly snacks to parties, and planning insulin doses ahead of time can help you manage fluctuations in blood sugar.

The Effects of Alcohol and Type 1 Diabetes

One of the biggest challenges for college students with T1D is navigating alcohol consumption. Alcohol can have a significant impact on blood sugar levels, and the effects can be unpredictable. Initially, alcohol can cause blood sugar to rise because of its carbohydrate content, especially in mixed drinks or sweet beverages. However, alcohol also impairs liver function, reducing the liver's ability to release glucose, which can result in delayed hypoglycemia (low blood sugar) several hours after drinking (American Diabetes Association, 2023).

Hypoglycemia is one of the most dangerous side effects of alcohol consumption for individuals with T1D. Alcohol-induced low blood sugar can go unnoticed because symptoms of hypoglycemia (e.g., dizziness, confusion, shakiness) can be similar to those caused by alcohol itself. For this reason, it's crucial to monitor blood glucose levels before and after drinking, eat a meal before consuming alcohol, and always have a source of glucose (such as glucose tablets or juice) nearby.

It's also important to have a plan for what to do if blood sugar levels drop while drinking. College students should never drink on an empty stomach and should always inform friends or roommates about their condition. Wearing a medical ID bracelet or carrying a diabetes alert card can be lifesaving in case of emergencies.

Strategies for Managing Diabetes in College

1. **Stay Organized**: Use planners or apps to track insulin doses, blood sugar levels, and meals.
2. **Practice Flexibility**: College life is unpredictable, so being able to adapt when things don't go as planned is key. This includes adjusting insulin doses or eating a snack if blood sugar drops unexpectedly.
3. **Social Support**: Surround yourself with people who understand

and respect your diabetes. Having a supportive social network can help you feel confident when navigating social situations.

4. **Communicate Your Needs**: Be open with friends, roommates, and college staff about your diabetes. This can help ensure your health is prioritized and that people are aware of what to do in case of a low blood sugar emergency.

While the college years present unique challenges for students with Type 1 Diabetes, they also offer opportunities for growth and independence. By staying organized, making informed choices, and using support networks, students can successfully manage their diabetes while enjoying the many experiences college life has to offer.

7

Relationships, Dating, and Type 1 Diabetes

Dear Diary: So, I went on a date tonight. It went well—until my blood sugar decided to crash mid-conversation. Cue awkward moment as I'm shoveling glucose tabs into my mouth. I'm pretty sure they think I'm a little weird now, but hey, at least they know I'm sweet... in more ways than one.

Managing Type 1 Diabetes (T1D) doesn't just involve taking care of your health—it also requires navigating relationships, both romantic and platonic. Whether you're dating, making new friends, or educating your family, communication and understanding are essential for a strong support system.

Dating with Type 1 Diabetes

When dating, it's important to share your T1D diagnosis at a time when the relationship feels comfortable and you trust the person. While it's not necessary to mention your condition immediately, being open about your diabetes helps avoid confusion if a situation arises, such as low blood sugar. A simple explanation like, *"I have Type 1 Diabetes, which means my body doesn't make insulin, so I need to manage my blood sugar with insulin and food"*, can ease the conversation and ensure your partner understands your needs (Steed et al., 2005).

Being honest can also help reduce any anxiety about how a partner may react. A supportive partner will respect your condition and work with you to ensure your health is managed without interfering with your relationship.

Educating Friends and Family

Explaining T1D to friends and family can help them support you better. Focus on the basics: what diabetes is, how you manage it, and what they can do in case of emergencies (e.g., recognizing signs of hypoglycemia). Providing resources or involving them in your care plan can strengthen relationships and ensure your loved ones know how to help if necessary.

Overcoming Stigma and Fear of Rejection

It's natural to fear rejection, especially when it comes to sharing something as personal as a chronic condition like Type 1 diabetes. The worry that others might not understand or might judge you can be overwhelming. However, it's important to remember that many people, once they learn about T1D, are more accepting than we often anticipate. The key to overcoming this fear lies in self-acceptance—your condition is just one part of who you are, but it does not define you. Embracing your diabetes and being open with others about it can actually foster stronger, more meaningful connections. When you're honest about your needs and experiences, it creates an opportunity for others to show empathy, understanding, and support. By breaking down the stigma surrounding diabetes, you not only help educate those around you but also build relationships that are grounded in trust and mutual respect. It's through this openness that you empower yourself and invite others to walk alongside you in a way that enriches both your life and theirs.

By educating others and communicating openly, managing T1D in relationships can be fulfilling and supportive. Building understanding within your social circles ensures that you have the support you need to thrive in your relationships.

8

What Happens When Things Go Wrong

Dear Diary: Well, today was one for the books... or diary. My blood sugar was playing ping-pong, and my CGM decided to take unapproved PTO. At least I didn't spill coffee on my meter... oh wait, I did.

Managing Type 1 Diabetes (T1D) can be a constant balancing act, and despite your best efforts, things don't always go as planned. Whether it's a blood sugar spike or a sudden drop, there are times when things can go wrong, and it's important to know how to troubleshoot and respond effectively.

Hypoglycemia: Low Blood Sugar

One of the most common challenges is hypoglycemia, or low blood sugar. Symptoms can include shakiness, sweating, confusion, irritability, or dizziness. It can happen for several reasons: taking too much insulin, skipping meals, or engaging in intense exercise without adjusting for insulin needs.

What to do: When you notice symptoms of hypoglycemia, the rule of thumb is to treat with 15 grams of fast-acting carbohydrates, such as glucose tablets, fruit juice, or regular soda (not diet). Wait 15 minutes, check your blood sugar again, and if it's still low, repeat the treatment.

Hyperglycemia: High Blood Sugar

On the flip side, hyperglycemia (high blood sugar) can also occur. Common causes include eating too many carbs without enough insulin, stress, or illness. Symptoms can include frequent urination, extreme thirst, fatigue, and blurred vision.

What to do: When your blood sugar is high, first check your insulin dose. If you've missed a dose or if you've overestimated your insulin needs, administer a correction dose. Drink plenty of water to help your body flush out excess sugar. If your blood sugar remains high and you develop symptoms of diabetic ketoacidosis (DKA)—such as nausea, vomiting, or deep, rapid breathing—seek medical help immediately (American Diabetes Association, 2023).

Insulin Pump or Injection Issues

If you use an insulin pump, it's important to check for issues like pump malfunctions or clogged tubing, which can prevent insulin delivery. If you're using injections, ensure you're rotating injection sites to avoid scar tissue buildup, which can affect insulin absorption.

What to do: Check your device and insulin sites regularly, and if you experience unexplained blood sugar highs or discomfort, troubleshoot by checking for air bubbles in the pump or poor absorption in injection areas. If problems persist, contact your healthcare provider or diabetes educator.

9

Celebrating Success and Living Your Best Life With Type 1

Dear Diary: Today was all about the little wins—checked my blood sugar (in range!), ate the right carbs, and didn't panic when my CGM beeped. Not life-changing, but hey, I'll take it. Baby steps, big wins.

Living with Type 1 Diabetes (T1D) requires ongoing management, but it's just as important to celebrate your successes, set future goals, and embrace the possibilities for a fulfilling life. While diabetes care can be challenging, focusing on achievements, learning from setbacks, and envisioning a positive future can help you thrive both physically and emotionally.

Celebrating Your Successes

In the midst of the day-to-day challenges, it can be easy to forget how far you've come. Managing T1D successfully—whether it's staying within your target blood sugar range, improving your A1C levels, or simply maintaining consistency in your routine—deserves recognition. Each small victory is a testament to your commitment, resilience, and ability to navigate the ups and downs of diabetes care.

Take time to reflect on what you've accomplished. Perhaps you've mastered carb counting, or you've figured out how to balance insulin and exercise. Maybe you've navigated stressful situations without letting your blood sugar get out of control. Celebrating these milestones can help you stay motivated and remind you that you are doing a great job.

One of the best ways to celebrate success is by rewarding yourself for staying on track with your diabetes management, whether through a special treat or a moment of relaxation. Positive reinforcement can create a sense of achievement and keep you feeling empowered in your journey.

Setting Future Goals

Once you've celebrated your successes, it's time to look forward and set new goals. Setting **SMART goals** (Specific, Measurable, Achievable, Relevant, Time-bound) can give you a clear path for continued improvement and help you stay focused.

Some examples of diabetes-related goals could include:

- **Improving your A1C**: If your goal is to lower your A1C, you might aim for a specific target over the next three to six months.
- **Enhancing your physical activity**: You may want to aim for a certain number of active minutes per week to improve your insulin sensitivity and overall well-being.
- **Mastering new technology**: If you're using an insulin pump or continuous glucose monitor (CGM), you might set a goal to learn more advanced features or fine-tune your settings.

It's also important to remember that goals are not just about numbers or results. They're about the process of self-improvement and staying engaged in your health. Goals should challenge you but be realistic enough to maintain your motivation and avoid burnout.

Living Your Best Life with Type 1 Diabetes

While managing T1D involves responsibility, it should never prevent you from living your best life. Many people with diabetes go on to achieve their dreams—whether in careers, relationships, travel, or fitness. **Your diagnosis does not limit your potential.** In fact, the skills you develop in managing diabetes—such as problem-solving, planning, and persistence—are transferable to many aspects of life.

Here are some tips for living your best life with Type 1 Diabetes:

1. **Stay connected to others**: Building a strong support network of family, friends, and peers who understand your journey can provide emotional support and encouragement.
2. **Embrace self-care**: Taking care of your mental health is just as important as managing your physical health. Engage in activities that make you feel good, whether it's meditation, spending time with loved ones, or pursuing a hobby.
3. **Be proactive**: Continue educating yourself about new diabetes technologies and treatment options. This not only empowers you but also helps you make informed decisions about your care.
4. **Find joy in the small moments**: While diabetes management can be demanding, it's important to remember that your quality of life is shaped by your mindset. Celebrate the simple things—whether it's a good blood sugar day or a fun activity with friends.

Success in managing Type 1 Diabetes isn't just about achieving perfect blood sugar control; it's about embracing the journey, setting meaningful goals, and living a full, rewarding life. By celebrating your accomplishments, setting realistic goals, and maintaining a positive outlook, you can navigate the challenges of diabetes management while living a life that is rich with potential and joy.

10

Conclusion: You've Got This!

Dear Diary: Okay, I think I'm finally getting the hang of this diabetes thing—turns out, all it takes is a little trial, error, and an occasional meltdown in the cereal aisle. I'm not saying I'm a pro yet, but I'm at least starting to feel like I'm playing in the minor leagues rather than just wandering around the field hoping someone hands me a bat. It's not always smooth sailing, but I'm pretty proud of my progress—and hey, if nothing else, I've gotten really good at making it look like I've got it all together.

Navigating life with Type 1 diabetes as a young adult is a unique journey filled with challenges and triumphs. From managing blood sugar levels and coordinating with a support team to balancing the demands of college and relationships, each step requires resilience, self-awareness, and a strong sense of empowerment. It's important to remember that while diabetes may shape your life, it does not define you. You are the one in control, and by taking ownership of your health, advocating for your needs, and embracing the support of those who care about you, you can lead a fulfilling and successful life. This journey is yours to shape—don't be afraid to take charge, ask for help when you need it, and celebrate the strength you discover along the way. Diabetes may be part of your story, but it is not the whole story, and you are capable of achieving great things!

11

Resources

American Diabetes Association. (2023). *Alcohol and diabetes.* Retrieved from https://www.diabetes.org

American Diabetes Association. (2023). *Hypoglycemia (low blood sugar) and hyperglycemia (high blood sugar).* Retrieved from https://www.diabetes.org

American Diabetes Association. (2023). *Living with diabetes.* Retrieved from https://www.diabetes.org

Anderson, B. J., et al. (2001). Psychological care of children and adolescents with diabetes. *Diabetes Care, 24*(6), 1326-1329.

Atkinson, M. A., Eisenbarth, G. S., & Michels, A. W. (2014). Type 1 diabetes. *Lancet, 383*(9911), 69-82. https://doi.org/10.1016/S0140-6736(13)60591-7

Cameron, F. J., et al. (2008). Diabetes-related distress in adolescents with type 1 diabetes: The role of family and school. *Pediatric Diabetes,*

9(5), 459-465.

Centers for Disease Control and Prevention (CDC). (2022). *Type 1 diabetes: Statistics and trends.* Retrieved from https://www.cdc.gov

Diabetes Technology Society. (2020). Using technology to manage type 1 diabetes. *Diabetes Technology & Therapeutics, 22*(2), 126-133. https://doi.org/10.1089/dia.2020.0015

Funnell, M. M., et al. (2009). The Diabetes Empowerment and Education Program (DEEP): A new approach to enhancing patient education. *Diabetes Care, 32*(7), 1127-1133.

Ludwig, D. S. (2002). The glycemic index: Implications for dietetics practice. *Journal of the American Dietetic Association, 102*(4), 511-514. https://doi.org/10.1016/S0002-8223(02)90204-6

Pouwer, F., et al. (2010). Diabetes-related emotional distress and health outcomes: A review of the literature. *Diabetes Research and Clinical Practice, 89*(2), 112-123.

Seidl, T., et al. (2020). Psychosocial aspects of diabetes: A review of interventions for promoting self-management. *Diabetes Spectrum, 33*(3), 204-211.

Steed, L., et al. (2005). Psychological impact of diabetes: The importance of relationships and support systems. *Diabetes Spectrum, 18*(4), 241-248.

Epilogue

If this book has helped you on your journey with Type 1 diabetes, I'd love to hear about it! Your feedback not only means the world to me, but it also helps others who may be searching for the support and guidance they need. If you found this guide helpful, please take a moment to leave a review on Amazon. Your words can make a real difference in helping others discover the resources they need to navigate their own path with confidence. Thank you for being part of this community, and for sharing your voice!